How to Think Like a

By Michael Mangold, MD

ISBN 9781520523293

Table of Contents

Preface to the First Edition

I came to Nicaragua originally to teach medical English to Nicaraguan medical students and intended to use this version as their textbook. My eventual goal is to revive Chairman Mao's concept of Barefoot Doctors and make quality medical and health care available to underserved areas of the world. It is not only a dream of mine but is the logical follow-up to my first non-profit endeavor The Medicine Cabinet, with which we collected, repackaged, and sent medications and medical equipment to areas of need. Our first shipment was sent to the Rwandan refugee camps in Zaire in 1994 and was one of the first humanitarian projects to arrive there since the tragedy was not recognized as a humanitarian crisis by developed nations for several months.

The world desperately needs kind, compassionate, and capable health care workers. Ironically (and sadly), this is the polar opposite of what is happening in the United States now where a "good doctor" is now defined by how quickly he or she charts. I personally do not want to go to the grave with the epitaph "Here lies Michael Mangold, a good doctor because he charted on time."

Michael Mangold, MD
San Juan del Sur, Nicaragua
September 2013

Preface to the Second Edition

Quite a bit has changed in medicine and my life since I first published this book. The United States has formally adopted ICD-10 for classifying diagnoses and so I have made the changes necessary to reflect this in the part of the book titled "Plan."

I have also "cleaned up" this book to improve "readability." Besides this, I want to integrate the intention of this book (medical education) with my overall goal of providing quality healthcare to underserved areas of the world and one way to do that is take advantage of the power of the internet to provide easy access to massive amounts of medical information.

While my goals have remained unchanged in the 3+ years since the initial publication, my life's situation has changed dramatically. I no longer live in Nicaragua. I am also semi-retired, thanks to the debilitating injuries I received in Managua trying to find my son Ben one Thanksgiving weekend.

Due to popular demand, I have added a section in "Additional Resources" concerning my diet and supplement recommendations.

As I tell readers of my blog, I hope that you will "Learn and Enjoy" the important things I have to say.

Michael Mangold MD
Chicago, IL USA
January 2017

What Is This Book?

How to Think Like a Doctor describes how a physician thinks. Whether you are a Medical Assistant student, a nursing student, a pre-med student, a new medical student, or even going into health care administration, you will benefit from discovering the process of how an M.D. or D.O. views any particular patient encounter and arrives at a diagnosis. The Diagnosis is key and ties together all of the other elements of the encounter so that a Plan can be formed to make the patient better. Improvement in health is why doctors do what they do and now you can gain an insight into that thought process.

Even if you are not a health care student or provider, How to Think Like a Doctor will make you a more knowledgeable patient. My best patients are those who become experts about their own bodies and their own medical and health issues. In addition to diseases, doctors address pain issues, mental health issues, dietary concerns, and even societal ills. Some physicians strive to make healthy people even better. So if you fall into any of these categories, you will benefit from this book.

"Let me recommend the best medicine in the world: a long journey, at a mild season, through a pleasant country, in easy stages."

---James Madison

Let's take President Madison's advice and enjoy this trip together. While medical school is a tough and frightening excursion, we are going to take the scenic route.

Introduction

You are a little scared. You do not feel "right" and now you are at the doctor's office to find out why and what can be done to make you feel better. The wait is long and the paperwork is even longer. A friendly nurse or Medical Assistant calls your name and leads you to a room. She gets a short story of why you are there, takes your vitals, and hands you a gown, reminding you to make sure the opening is in the back. As she leaves, she states that the "doctor will be right in."

You know the rest of the story. The physician comes in, reads what the nurse wrote, goes over the vital signs, asks you a few questions, and then does a physical exam (which are very focused and brief these days). When he is done, he heads to the door, tells you he will be right back, and in that in the meantime, "you can get dressed now." When he comes back he says you have this or that condition (diagnosis), he may want to run some tests, and then hands you a prescription to treat your condition.

"Any questions?"

Yes. What just happened? How did the doctor do that (arrive at his diagnosis and plan)?

By the end of How to Think Like a Doctor, you will know the answer to these questions. I am going to lead you through the process or the steps good doctors follow in the "art and science of Medicine" so that you will be well-informed, well-armed, and wiser for the effort. If you are a healthcare student, the patient-physician encounter will no longer be that "black box" that occurs between the time the patient walks into an exam room and when she walks out. Nursing students will appreciate discovering the difference between how nurses and doctors think. And pre-med and medical students: well, this is a great introduction to the practice of medicine and will hopefully make your didactic studies come alive.

Another hope is that budding health care administrators will also learn to appreciate the job that a good physician does and to realize that not everything in medicine is rote and quantifiable. There really is an "art" side to it.

"Medicine is not only a science; it is also an art. It does not consist of compounding pills and plasters; it deals with the very processes of life, which must be understood before they may be guided."

---Paracelsus

How To Think Like a Doctor

Fortunately, medical training has already given me a template for teaching you how to think like a doctor. That template is the doctor's note. A doctor's note can be hand-written, dictated, or generated through an Electronic Medical Record ("EMR"). The standard, almost universal charting method is called a "SOAP Note" and I will show you how the broader categories of the SOAP Note reflect more specific "doctor think." This acronym stands for:

S = Subjective or what the patient, friends, and/or family tells the doc.

O = Objective or what a physician finds via a physical examination and/or test results.

A = Assessment or what a physician thinks is going on with a patient. The assessment will include at least one diagnosis.

P = Plan. Now that we know what is going on, what are we going to do about it?

Ideally, a third-party person should be able to pick up a well-written note and follow the physician's thinking. The conclusion (Diagnosis and Plan) should follow logically from the antecedent premises (History and Physical). This book will use a case study to illuminate the facts I present in this book, explaining at each point of the template how it relates to you. Doctors love case studies. A case study is a summary of an actual patient encounter usually presented in the format I am teaching here. We will be following Mrs. G (a real patient of mine) and I will end each major area in this book with the relevant parts of her story: my actual SOAP Note from that encounter.

The full case study is repeated without breaks in the SUMMARY section of this book. As a small exercise, read it now before moving on, then re-read it when you are done with the book. If I have done my job well you will note the growth you have made by learning "how a doctor thinks."

About the words used in this book: speech and writing reflect thought processes. Physicians use words specific to medicine called medical jargon or what I call "med-speak." Look up any word or phrase you are not familiar with in the GLOSSARY towards the end of this book. Doctors are also good at creating acronyms and the most frequently used acronyms in medicine are officially accepted by the medical community. Lastly, because of the vast amount of information a physician must acquire, a lot of it can be summarized and remembered through the use of mnemonics.

How To Think Like a Doctor presents, explains, and gives examples using a standard doctor's SOAP note as the template:

Subjective
A. Chief Complaint
B. History of Present Illness
C. Past Medical History
D. Family History
E. Social History

Objective
A. Vital Signs
B. General

C. Mental Status

D. Focused Physical Exam vs. General or Full Physical Exam

E. Physical exam by organ system

F. Abnormal findings

G. Test results: what normal and abnormal results mean

Assessment

A. The Differential Diagnosis

B. A Presumptive Diagnosis

C. The Definitive Diagnosis

The Plan

A. The importance of Medical Decision-Making

B. Medical Necessity

C. Medications

D. Therapies

E. Referrals/Consultations

F. Follow-up

SUBJECTIVE

"A doctor who cannot take a good history and a patient who cannot give one are in danger of giving and receiving bad treatment.

---Author Unknown

A patient goes to the doctor's office for a reason. Whether he called first or walked-in off the street, there has to be a purpose for his visit and that purpose is called the Chief Complaint ("CC"). Besides demographics (name, age, address, insurance coverage, etc.), a lot of the initial paperwork and questioning will center on expanding the Chief Complaint. The ability to gather details will depend on the training of the staff member the patient is dealing with at any given moment. The receptionist will often just write down the

Chief Complaint, perhaps even getting a time of symptom onset. An M.A. will fill in more of the details, and a nurse will dig deep and pull out even more relevant information. It really surprises me, too, when I go into a room and the patient tells me things he did not mention to the nurse or M.A. By the time a physician steps in the room, she has probably already read the nursing notes and now her questions will be even more precise and focused.

Chief Complaint: Why are you at the doctor's office today?

Case Study: A 62 year-old woman (Mrs. G) calls the doctor's clinic and says she wants to be seen for a rash that is getting worse.
What is her Chief Complaint? Worsening rash.

History of Present Illness ("HPI")

This part of the History deals with details of the Chief Complaint. At this point, the physician knows only why the patient wants to be seen and maybe how long the symptoms have been present. A good HPI will address the following concerns:

What are your symptoms?

When did they start?

Have you done anything yourself to help your symptoms? If so, did it work?

Is there anything that makes the symptoms worse? Better?

If the Chief Complaint is not related to pain, are there any pain issues that need to be addressed.

Case Study: Mrs. G describes a "rash" that started one week ago on the skin of her abdomen. It is very itchy. She describes the rash as "little red bumps" that have spread from her abdomen, across her lower back, and even down her pelvic region to the top of the front of her thighs.

She explains that she has used over-the-counter ("OTC") Caladryl Lotion which does lessen the itching for a few hours but has failed to halt the spread of the rash. Cold water also works for itch relief but only for the duration of application.

As an aside, Mrs. G states that her right hip hurts when she walks any significant distance.

The Pain Assessment follows. The mnemonic for The Pain Assessment is "PQRST":
P = Provocative events (what provokes the pain)
What causes the pain?
What makes it better?

Worse?

Q = Quality

What does it feel like?

Is it sharp?

Dull?

Stabbing?

Burning?

Crushing?

R = Radiates

Where does the pain start?

To where does the pain radiate, if at all?

Is it in one place?

Does it go anywhere else?

Did it start elsewhere and now localized to one spot?

S = Severity

How severe is the pain on a scale of 1 - 10?

Younger children can use an illustrated pain scale such as the "Wong-Baker Pain Scale" which is fairly accurate and reproducible:

Wong-Baker FACES Pain Rating Scale

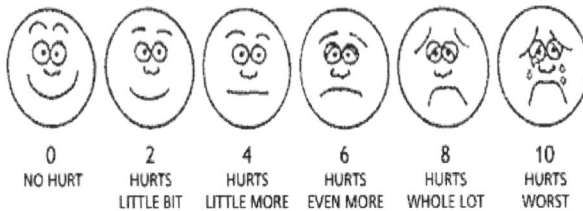

0	2	4	6	8	10
NO HURT	HURTS LITTLE BIT	HURTS LITTLE MORE	HURTS EVEN MORE	HURTS WHOLE LOT	HURTS WORST

From Wong D.L., Hockenberry-Eaton M., Wilson D., Winkelstein M.L., Schwartz P.: Wong's Essentials of Pediatric Nursing, ed. 6, St. Louis, 2001, p. 1301. Copyrighted by Mosby, Inc. Reprinted by permission.

T = Time

When did the pain start?

How long did it last?

Is it constant or intermittent?

Case Study: Mrs. G says the pain in her right hip occurs only after walking at least 6 city blocks. Resting makes it feel better as does taking OTC ibuprofen. Ice has no effect.

The pain is described as "dull" and does not radiate anywhere else. It gets progressively worse the further she walks and can start out as low as a "4" on a scale of 0-10 and end up debilitating her when it gets to an "8". She first noticed the pain about 2 years ago, before her husband's retirement, but it is much more noticeable now that they spend more time walking together.

Past Medical History ("PMH")

When a patient is seen for the first time, the PMH becomes a part of the permanent chart. A physician can review it and determine if anything in the past could contribute to the Chief Complaint. Working forward, a good

PMH also helps finalize a Diagnosis. During subsequent visits, a review of a patient's PMH also focuses the doctor's attention on the possibility that her own previous treatments may contribute to the current complaint.

Have you had these symptoms before? If so, what were you diagnosed with?

Do you have any chronic illnesses? Are you taking any medications and if so, what are they?

Has there been a recent medication change?

Have you had any recent travel away from home? If so, when and to where?

Are you taking any OTC medications? Any supplements?

Do you have any environmental allergies?

Do you have any medication allergies?

Have you had any prior surgeries?

For females: how many times have you been pregnant and how many children do you have? Were they uncomplicated pregnancies? Were there any problems during delivery or any postpartum complications? Are you still menstruating? When was the date of your last menstrual period? Could you be pregnant?

Case Study: while Mrs. G states that she obviously has had rashes in the past, this is the first time for her that one has lasted this long and it is worrying her. Her only diagnosed medical condition is hypertension (HTN) and she takes Lisinopril once-a-day which does help control her blood pressure. She has never had any serious side-effects from it and as far as she knows, does not have any drug allergies. She is also allergic to ragweed but at this time of year (early Spring), she has not had any problems. During allergy season, she self-medicates with OTC Loratadine.

Since her husband's retirement two years ago, the couple bought a house on the east coast of Florida. They just returned to the Midwest to visit relatives last week, about the same time as the onset of the rash. They enjoy each others company and spend their leisure time going for walks, swimming in the ocean, and eating out. Mrs. G has never felt better in her relationship with her husband and domestic violence is not now nor ever has been a concern.

She has two healthy grown children, one boy and one girl. At 45 years of age, she had a cholecystectomy to remove her gallbladder. The same year she had an elective hysterectomy. Because her uterus was removed, she does not know precisely when she started menopause but believes she had peri-menopausal symptoms about 10 years ago.

Family History ("FH")

Is anyone else in your family sick with the same symptoms?
Are there any chronic illnesses in your family?
Are your parents still alive? If not, what are the causes of death?
Are your siblings still alive? If not, what are the causes of death?

Social History ("SH")

With whom do you live?
Are your living arrangements safe?
Do you wear a seatbelt?

Are there any guns in the house?

Do you feel safe at home? Never ask this in front of another family member.

Do you smoke, drink, do drugs?

Do you work outside of the home? If so, doing what?

Are you exposed to any noxious chemicals at home or work?

Are you pregnant? (For fertile females).

Do you have any pets?

Case Study: No one else in her family has the same symptoms, including her husband. Her mother had lupus ("SLE") and died of complications related to a cerebrovascular accident ("CVA") or stroke at 85 years old. Her father had Type II Diabetes Mellitus ("DMII") (or Adult-Onset Diabetes), heart disease, emphysema, and died of an Acute Myocardial Infarction ("AMI") or heart attack when he was

68. Mrs. G believes that most of his problems were due to poor lifestyle choices including smoking 1-2 packs of cigarettes a day for 50 years and eating a poor diet.

The patient started smoking cigarettes when she was 15 but quit when she got pregnant with her first child at 22 years old. She does have a history of marijuana use during her "hippie days" but feels it was not an addiction. She does drink socially but cannot remember the last time she got drunk. She had been a stay-at-home mom for 30 years and once her second child left home, she volunteered at church and at a local assisted living facility ("ALF"). She has no known long-term exposure to any noxious chemicals "unless you count household cleaners." Up until two years ago, Mr. and Mrs. G had two cats and a dog. Since then, the dog died and the cats were given away to friends prior to going to Florida.

That ends the Subjective part of the encounter. Take a moment and think about all of the information the physician and staff have gathered at this point. In an ideal world, each encounter would include all of the aspects presented here. In reality, the staff and doctor may not obtain so many details due to time constraints. One adage in medical school is that 80% of the information needed to make the correct diagnosis is in the history-taking. It is amazing how a good history can narrow down the possibilities. And also point you in the right direction.

OBJECTIVE

"A good physical examination separates the men from the boys, and the women from the girls."

---Michael Mangold, MD

A good clinician is worth his weight in gold. Kind of. In reality, clinical skills do not pay while medical decision-making does. In spite of that, I believe that performing an appropriate, thorough, and accurate physical examination is a key component of the physician/patient relationship. A physician needs an adequate education in anatomy and physiology ("A&P") and most importantly, needs to know the difference between "normal" and "abnormal." A big advantage is that humans are bilaterally symmetrical meaning that we have left and right sides that appear to be equal. A few exceptions occur with some internal organs such as heart and pancreas but for the most part, if you can visualize it, it has a bilateral counterpart.

The physical examination uses certain tools to discover areas of abnormality and also to reinforce what is normal. The most important tools are the doctor's senses: does she look right? Are there any peculiar smells? Is that the way speech is supposed to sound? Is that the way joints sound when a limb is moved? Does this hurt to touch it? Is the skin warm and dry, etc?

A physician can tell a great deal just by observing the patient. However, an investigation into pathology requires certain other tools. These include a sphygmomanometer for measuring blood pressure, a light to check pupils and other areas, a stethoscope for listening to heart, lung, abdominal, and other sounds, and a reflex hammer to check neurological function. These are the basics that I carry in my doctor's bag. There are other tools of course, and some of them are used only for specific circumstances. For example, a UV light is used to see if a rash is caused by a fungus and an ophthalmoscope is used to check the back of the eyeball. As with any tool, these require a mentor to show proper technique (think of your dad teaching you to hammer in a nail). And, as with any tool, perfect practice makes perfect.

The physical examination can be approached in several ways. A focused exam will guide you to the anatomical area under discussion.

For example, the doctor could merely look at Mrs. G's rash and try to make a diagnosis from there. Unfortunately, in our rushed approach to medicine these days, more and more patient encounters include just focused exams and physicians are missing opportunities to care for the whole patient. Because health care providers are often paid on an unspoken quota basis, this approach is understandable but still lamentable.

A thorough physical examination will move in one of two predictable ways: either from body part-to-body part or from organ system-to-organ system. My own preference is a mixture of the two: I move head-to-toe (well, actually it starts with a general picture of overall patient health) and I tie up loose ends by addressing the organ systems. This approach reminds me what to check for at each visit and hopefully the important findings will not be overlooked. In this book, as I move head-to-toe, I will point out some of the organ systems covered in each body part. In the "Summary" towards the end of the book, I will explain the importance of the organ system approach.

Vital Signs ("VS")

Heart Rate ("HR")

Blood Pressure ("BP")

Respiratory Rate ("RR")

Temperature ("T")

Oxygen Saturation ("SaO_2")

Height

Weight

Body Mass Index ("BMI") for adults and older children

Growth Chart for children

General ("GEN")

Does the patient appear well or ill? Is he overweight or underweight? Is she physically in shape? Does the patient appear to be free of pain? Is there anything in the first impression that raises a cause for concern?

Mental Status ("MS" or "MSE")

A quick device used to report a patient's level of awareness and ability to understand questions. A physician's report will usually abbreviate this to "A, A, Ox3, in NAD" which means "awake, alert, oriented to person, place, and time, and in no acute distress." This quick check is part of the Psychiatric System ("Psych") which is covered in more detail later.

Head, Eyes, Ears, Nose, and Throat ("HEENT")

This examination requires a flashlight to document pupillary response to light. Examination of the back of the eyeball requires an ophthalmoscope while visualization of the inside of the ear requires an otoscope. Physical traits that are grossly observable include whether there are any skull abnormalities, whether the eyeballs are symmetrical and move together, and whether facial movements are normal and symmetric. Hearing can be tested during this exam as well as vision with an eye chart.

Neck

Observe movement of the head. Does it move normally or does the patient "guard" his movements? Feel (palpate) the front and back of the neck. The front of the body is known as the anterior while the back of the body is known as its posterior. A part of the body above another is known as "superior" while the lower part is "inferior." During this exam, we move from superior to inferior (except when we get to the psychiatric part!). Palpating (feeling) the anterior neck checks on the thyroid gland which is part of the Endocrine System. Checking the neck for the presence of lymph nodes is also part of the Lymphatic System.

Case study: Mrs. G is a well-nourished, obese female. Vital signs show a heart rate of 78 beats per minute ("BPM"), a BP of 142/88 mmHg, a RR of 16/minute, and a temperature of 98.8 degrees Fahrenheit. Her height is 63 inches and her weight is 195 pounds giving her a BMI of 34.5.

The patient is A, A, Ox3, and in some mild distress due to itching. She is scratching at her lower abdomen. Head is normocephalic ("NCAT"), atraumatic (normal shape and without evidence of trauma). Pupils are equally round and reactive to light and accommodation ("PERRLA"). Extra-ocular movements are intact ("EOM-I"): in other words they move normally and in tandem with each other. Sclerae (the whites of the eyes) are white. While Mrs. G wears corrective lenses, vision was not tested.

Ears are clear bilaterally and hearing is grossly normal. No nasal discharge is present and nasal mucus membranes are moist. Pharynx is clear; uvula rises midline. Teeth show normal signs of aging but there are no apparent tooth fractures

Neck is supple with a full range-of-motion ("FROM"). The posterior neck is nontender and without spasms. Palpation of the anterior neck is without thyromegaly (enlarged thyroid) or masses. There is no cervical lymphadenopathy.

Thorax (that part of the body from the neck to the abdomen)

a. Upper back

Examination of the back should include visualization of the spine to see if it is straight or not and palpation of the muscles to check for areas of tenderness and spasm. Two conditions that can be visualized by looking at the spine include kyphosis (over-curvature of the thoracic spine) and scoliosis (curved side-to-side).

Other organ systems we check on during the upper back exam include MSK and NEURO.

<u>b. Chest</u>

Look for symmetry and make sure the left and right chest rise equally with each breath. Look for obvious deformities including pectus carinatum (also known as "pigeon chest"). A breast exam would include a more detailed approach than I can give here. In Mrs. G's case, since her Chief Complaint did not contain any symptoms associated with breast diseases, I did not do a breast exam. That was "deferred" to a later date.

<u>c. Heart/Cardiovascular System ("CV")</u>

A doctor can percuss or tap the chest to check for heart size. Some heart problems can also be visualized. Auscultation of the heart and lungs with a stethoscope is mandatory in every exam. Another way to check heart function is to look for edema in the patient's feet and ankles.

When we check for edema, we are also examining the Derm System.

d. Lungs/Pulmonary System ("PULM")

Percuss and auscultate. Another check for lung function is to look for cyanosis or a bluish discoloration of fingertips or around the mouth.

Again, a check of the skin for cyanosis means that we checked the Derm System.

Abdomen/Gastrointestinal System ("GI"): that part of the front (anterior) of the body between the thorax and the pelvis. I include the lower back in this part of the exam since I am "down there anyway."

Since abdominal findings such as bowel sounds can be affected by pressing on the belly, a physician will first look at it carefully, noting any bloating, masses, or asymmetry. Secondly, he will auscultate, listening for the presence of bowel sounds and whether they are of normal pitch and located in all areas (the four quadrants). At that point, the abdomen will be palpated and even percussed.

Lower back

Examination of the lumbar or lower back is the same as the thoracic back exam. The doc will look for normal and abnormal curves. On yourself, note that the lower back naturally has a curve anteriorly (towards the front of the body). This is called lordosis and straightening of the curve is abnormal. Scoliosis can affect the lumbar spine, too. The physician will feel the muscles surrounding the spine ("paralumbar" muscles), noting any spasms and tenderness. It is also possible to sometimes feel protruding disks between lumbar vertebrae, or intervertebral masses.

Case Study: Upper back shows mild kyphosis. Spine is otherwise midline and parathoracic muscles are without tenderness or spasms. There is no nipple retraction on visual inspection but a full breast examination is deferred.

Heart has a regular rate and rhythm ("RRR") and is without murmurs or rubs. No edema is noted.

Lungs are clear to auscultation ("CTA") bilaterally and there is good respiratory excursion. No cyanosis is noted.

Abdomen is non-distended ("ND") and bowel sounds are normoactive ("BSNA") and present in all quadrants. Abdomen is soft and nontender to palpation. No masses or hepatosplenomegaly ("HSM") are present. She does have a rash present on the skin of her lower abdomen which will be covered in more detail in "DERM."

Lumbar spine is straight and non-tender. There is minor tenderness along the right paralumbar muscles but no spasms are palpable. She has limited range-of-motion ("ROM") to forward flexion (bending forward) at the waist, limited by both an increase of pain and decreased flexibility.

Did you follow all of that? I hope so and I hope that you can start to see that charting reflects how a doctor thinks. If you had a difficult time with the last part of the Case Study, look up each of the med-speak words you are not familiar with in the "Glossary" and try it again. I worked in the ER for almost 20 years and speaking/writing like this became so routine I could literally do it in my sleep.

Pelvis
a. Hips
b. Genitourinary System ("GU")
c. Lower GI System (rectum and anus)

This is one part of the physical examination that many physicians skip when it is deemed unnecessary. Good charting will reflect that the doctor thought about this area but did not do a full exam. For example, this is another area which is often "deferred." Obviously, if a patient comes in for complaints related to the genitals, a genital exam would be mandatory. In Mrs. G's case, her rash had spread from her lower abdomen to that part of her pelvic region known as the "inguinal area" so even just a cursory look there was important.

Case Study: Visual inspection shows spread of her abdominal rash to her inguinal areas bilaterally. A full description of the rash is found under "DERM."

Right lateral hip is tender to palpation. She has FROM of the right lower extremity ("LE") at the hip with increasing pain to lateral abduction. The right anterior-superior iliac crest ("ASIC" = top of hip) is elevated anteriorly about 3 cm above the left.

Of note, she does have a single right inguinal lymph node, about 1cm round, which is tender, soft, and mobile.

Musculoskeletal System ("MSK")

A good doctor will note limitations in movement of each of the major joints (shoulders, elbows, wrists, and knees) and if there are concerns about any specific joint, will do specialized testing, comparing right vs. left and noting any discrepancies. A goniometer is a device she can use to measure ROM in degrees. It looks like a mathematician's protractor with arms.

In Mrs. G's case, the ROM of her head and legs were already assessed as well as the alignment of her spine. A good MSK exam will also note gait and strength. Like most other human physical attributes, strength can be measured and physicians will grade it on a scale of 0-5, with 0 being a totally flaccid muscle group and a 5 being full strength and function. Forearm and hand strength can be measure with a manometer which a patient squeezes. It is useful for measuring grip strength over time as well as for comparing left vs. right.

Case Study: MSK exam shows FROM of her head and shoulders. Lumbar spine is straight and non-tender. There is minor tenderness along the right paralumbar muscles but no spasms are palpable. She has limited ROM to forward flexion at the waist. Right hip is tender laterally with decreased ROM to abduction of her right lower extremity. Right ASIC is elevated compared to the left. Gait is occasionally hesitant due to pain in her right hip but otherwise normal. Grip strength in both hands is strong (+5/5) and she is able to stand on her tip-toes.

Skin/Dermatological System ("DERM")

You can't hide all of your skin and a good physician will quickly do a skin examination just by looking at you. A more detailed or focused skin exam should follow if the Chief Complaint warrants it. Many systemic diseases have dermatological or skin manifestations (for example, SLE has a characteristic "butterfly rash" on the face). On the other hand, many rashes are localized and have outside (exogenous) causes and no underlying systemic disease. To complicate things even more, different people may present with different skin manifestations of the same disease and rashes may change characteristics over time. In general, a quick exam will note the color of the skin, the hydration of the skin, and any abnormalities. Skin color may be normal (and that depends on the patient's ethnicity), pale, cyanotic or blue, or reddened. Especially notable in mucus membranes such as the mouth but also noticeable in the eyes, skin may be dry or well-hydrated. Other abnormalities include edema, rashes, the presence of lesions, or signs of infection.

Case Study: Mrs. G's skin is warm and dry; mucus membranes are moist. There is no cyanosis or edema. She has a red, papular rash from the skin of the lower quadrants of her abdomen bilaterally which radiates into both inguinal areas. Papules are 1-2mm round and raised.

Endocrine/Lymphatic system ("ENDO"; "LYMPH")

I put these two together since they are usually brief and tend to be covered in other body part examinations. For example, diabetes is an endocrine disease and dehydration is one physical manifestation of this disease. A doctor checks on lymph nodes in the neck, the inguinal area, and sometimes the axillae (armpits). Blood disorders and cancers can affect the lymphatic system as well and the specialists who care for these patients are called "Hematologist/Oncologists" and the system is "HEME/ONC." Instead of a separate Lymphatic system category, some physicians will give it that label.

Case Study: As noted previously, the patient's mucus membranes are moist and she is well-hydrated. There is no cervical lymphadenopathy, one right inguinal lymph node, and no enlarged thyroid or thyroid masses can be palpated.

Neurological system ("NEURO")

Many physicians will combine the neurological and psychiatric examinations under one heading called "NEURO-PSYCH." A large part of my training is in psychiatry and while in the end, psychiatric problems are really neurologic issues, I feel they deserve separate attention, at least in the primary care setting.

The neurological exam begins with examination of gait. We all know what constitutes a normal and an abnormal walk. Problems with gait can be due to many causes such as rheumatological and musculoskeletal disorders as well as neurological disorders. At this point, observations need to be made and charted while the sorting out process occurs later during the Assessment and Plan parts.

After observing the gait, a good doctor will observe problems with eye movements and speech. There are twelve sets of nerves in the brainstem called the Cranial Nerves and they are abbreviated CNN I-XII. The first cranial nerve is related to your sense of smell (olfaction) and is rarely ever tested in the primary care setting. If a physician takes the time to check on the other cranial nerves, she will run you through a set of testing that seems silly at the time. For example, tracking your eye movements; whether you can smile and raise your shoulders; and even puff out your cheeks. If this is even done, she will abbreviate the note as "CNN II-XII were tested and are grossly intact."

We all also know what normal speech is. Speech disorders have several causes including learning disorders, neurological disorders (such as stroke), and musculoskeletal problems. An example of the latter is people with Down Syndrome who have weak tongue muscles.

Another part of the neuro exam is a check on balance. Balance is controlled by the posterior-inferior part of your brain called the cerebellum. The cerebellum can be adversely affected by strokes and noxious chemicals such as alcohol and certain drugs. Think of the testing a cop does on suspected drunk drivers. Heel-to-toe walking is one example.

Case Study: As stated previously, Mrs. G's gait is hesitant due to pain in her right hip. Cranial nerves II-XII were tested and are grossly intact. Speech has a normal cadence and reflects appropriate thought content. Balance is good and she is able to perform heel-to-toe walking without difficulty.

Psychiatric exam ("PSYCH")

Orientation is the first part of the psychiatric examination and as explained in GEN, a normal patient's level of awareness, orientation to person, place, and time, and level of distress is abbreviated to A, A, Ox3, in NAD (no acute distress). Level of awareness can be affected by brain disorders, mood disorders, alcohol and other drugs of abuse (ADOA), and even time of day or night. Distress is a sign of inner turmoil and can be caused by such factors as anxiety and pain and even withdrawal from addictive drugs. Psychiatric, neurologic, and physical factors all contribute to a person's state of health and should be noted in the chart.

Thought content is reflected in a patient's speech. Is the speech rushed? Is the patient logical and does what she say flow appropriately from the current situation? Are there any threats of harming one's self or someone else?

Case Study: The patient is A, A, Ox3, and in mild distress secondary to itchiness. She is not anxious but is concerned about her illness. Her mood is appropriate to the situation, not sad, and she expresses no suicidal or homicidal ideations.

Test Results

"Treat the patient, not the X-ray.

---James M. Hunter

If testing is done in the clinic, the results go here. The federal government allows clinics to perform a certain number of tests called "CLIA-Waived Tests." A physician will pay the government to run a limited number of tests in-house and in turn, the government ensures that the tests are accurate and performed appropriately. More can be found at their website listed in the "References" section of this book.

Common CLIA-Waived tests include urine pregnancy, rapid strep, urinalysis hemoglobin, and blood sugar tests. Testing itself is usually performed by the M. A. or nurse and results recorded immediately. Some physicians will do microscopic testing and even perform x-rays in the clinic although these are becoming rarer.

If the physician thinks that testing is medically necessary, he will order the tests and note them in the chart. He should also justify why the tests are necessary. This justification is important in our health care environment because the government and insurance companies will scrutinize these orders before reimbursing for the tests. If the doctor is part of a hospital system, he can write the orders and the patient theoretically has the choice of where she wants them performed. More often than not, it is within the hospital system itself.

Case Study: Phlebotomy (blood draw) was performed and the tube sent to lab for a rheumatology panel because of the patient's right hip pain. I also ordered a right hip x-ray to check for degenerative changes as a cause of the pain, and a low back x-ray because of her tenderness and limited range of motion to forward flexion. Results were pending by the end of her visit.

ASSESSMENT

"Of two equivalent theories or explanations, all other things being equal, the simpler one is to be preferred."

---William of Ockham

"When you hear hoofbeats, think horses, not zebras."

---Medical school adage

"Watch out for zebras."

---Michael Mangold, M.D.

The World Health Organization (WHO) devised a list of diagnoses which makes it easier for physicians to narrow down the possibilities. Physicians get reimbursed by insurance companies, Medicaid, and

Medicare based on two sets of codes: the ICD code and the Current Procedural Terminology ("CPT") Code. The latter is a copyrighted set of codes devised and published by the American Medical Association ("AMA"). Every time a provider uses a CPT code, the AMA gets its cut.

Some pathologies are easy to diagnose; some are not. There are three levels of certainty when it comes to making a diagnosis: the "Differential Diagnosis" which is a list of possible diagnoses. The "Presumptive Diagnosis" which is the working conclusion for most patient encounters. It is the physician's best guess of what is ailing a patient based on the elements of the History and Physical during a particular encounter (although most doctors will not explain that it is a guess). And lastly, there is the "Definitive Diagnosis" which occurs after all of the test results are in.

The Differential Diagnosis

What are all of the possible things this could be? I can best explain this by going over our Case Study and my thinking process involved in this example. For this particular encounter, we have arrived at two major problems: her rash and her hip pain; and several minor problems, including obesity, lower back pain, and hypertension. When I first started medical school, we used a process of rule-outs ("R/O") to arrive at a definitive diagnosis. Rule-outs are no longer accepted by the powers-that-be but every good doctor keeps this process in the back of his mind while strategizing a treatment plan.

Case Study: Here is my list of the primary rule-outs for Mrs. G:

A. Rash (dermatitis)

1. Contact dermatitis

2. Skin manifestation of an allergic reaction

3. Rash caused by ocean-dwelling organisms

4. Atypical lupus rash

B. Right hip pain

1. Pain in hip

2. Soft tissue pain

3. Pain caused by rheumatoid arthritis

4. Pain caused by osteoarthritis

5. Pain is secondary to osteoporosis

Here is my list of secondary diagnoses, which may or may not be related to the primary diagnoses:

1. Mild Hypertension

2. Low Back Pain

A patient can have more than one diagnosis for the same complaint especially if one of the diagnoses is a general description such as "pain." She does have pain in her hip. Now, what is causing that pain? Some doctors will treat the pain and never look into causes.

The Presumptive Diagnosis

Practically speaking, treatments can be the same for several diagnoses. For Mrs. G, I knew that a topical steroid ointment would alleviate her itching whether her definitive diagnosis was 1, 2, or 3 under "Rash." I also knew that her hip pain would be relieved by non-steroidal anti-inflammatory drugs ("NSAIDs") whether it was caused by rheumatoid arthritis, osteoarthritis, or osteoporosis.

The Definitive Diagnosis

The lab and x-ray results came in about 3 days after I saw Mrs. G in the clinic. Current EHR's will allow a physician to add an Addendum to report the results and some EHR's are integrated with the labs and radiology departments so that the results are put directly in the charts. For Mrs. G, the rheumatology panel was negative for any autoimmune disease such as lupus while her hip x-ray showed changes consistent with osteoarthritis. Based on her history of swimming in the ocean off of the coast of Florida prior to developing the rash, I called an Emergency Room in Port St. Lucie, Florida and asked if there were any water-borne outbreaks going on at the time. They advised me that the organisms responsible for "swimmer's itch" had been prevalent for the last month. So I gave her the Definitive Diagnosis of "Rash caused by ocean-dwelling organisms." The ER doc also gave me information on how to treat the rash.

Her second Definitive Diagnosis was "Pain caused by osteoarthritis." I could now formulate a treatment plan that was more specific to each one those diagnoses.

THE PLAN

A. The importance of Medical Decision-Making

Because of my experiences running my own clinic, I came to understand that medical decision-making is where a good physician really shines. Especially at the primary care level, huge forces pull at doctors to do or not do certain things. Consider the tensions involved: hospital systems want physicians to use the hospital's labs, radiology departments, specialized therapy groups, and specialists. The government wants to eliminate unnecessary testing and referrals. Private insurance companies want to honor their promises (contracts) to their enrollees while saving money. Professional organizations want to promote their constituency. Most importantly, patients want to get better.

Books have been written on how to be a better decision-maker. There are even societies and journals that claim to do the same: http://www.smdm.org. Here is my dilemma: do I spend up to $50 to buy a book that I may or may not need and is my time best spent looking up ways to make the best decisions or should I focus on patient care instead?

B. Medical Necessity

How does a doctor justify his plans? The answer to that is determining what is medically necessary to get the patient better. Medical Necessity is the driving force behind current medical decision-making. Much of that "necessity" is defined by reimbursements. What will or will not the government and insurance companies pay for? The Centers for Medicare and Medicaid even have forms that physicians need to fill out before they will pay for certain services and goods: http://www.cms.gov/Medicare/CMS-Forms/CMS-Forms/CMS-Forms-List.html.

Based on a quality history and physical examination, what further studies are necessary? Can a Definitive Diagnosis be made at that particular encounter? If not, what further studies, referrals, and/or consultations will help the doc arrive there? Can he use the diagnosis to justify certain therapies, including medications? Is it justifiable to do nothing at all? "Watch & Wait" is also a part of some plans.

C. Medications

Allopathic physicians (M.D.) and Osteopathic physicians (D.O.) prescribe medications. Before a medication is prescribed, a good doctor will ask himself or herself the following questions:

1. Based on the diagnosis or diagnoses, what is the best medication for this person?

2. Does the patient have any drug allergies? Will this medication precipitate an allergic reaction in this patient?

3. What are the medication side-effects? Can this patient tolerate the side-effects? Do the benefits of the medication exceed the side-effects in this particular case?

4. Is the patient taking other medications that will interact with this one? Conversely, will this new medication help alleviate some of the side-effects of other medications?

5. Is there a generic equivalent that is less expensive? What are the advantages of the non-generic medicine compared to generic alternatives? Will the patient's insurance pay for the medication or is the patient responsible for a large co-pay or is she even self-pay?

6. If there are multiple pathologies, will one medication help both? Make one worse? Make two better and one worse? Or are more medications needed?

7. On what information do I base my decision? Did I read it in a good peer-reviewed article? Did I see an ad on TV or professional

magazine, or have it explained to me by a pharmaceutical rep at a specialty conference? Did the patient suggest a particular medication?

8. Lastly, am I free from bias in making this recommendation?

For a lot of reasons, medicine in this country is driven by prescriptions. It's not just because of the political influence of the large pharmaceutical companies either. Insurance companies, for example, encourage doctors to write prescriptions as evidence that patients are seen. Patients themselves expect prescriptions from their physicians. I had a patient once who came to see me for several problems, including obesity, anxiety, and knee pain. After an hour of history taking and a full examination, I told her that all of her issues could be addressed by simple measures. If she lost weight, I explained (I also discussed weight loss plans with her), her knee pain would lessen if not go away completely. In the meantime, she could take OTC NSAIDs as needed. I advised her to take a yoga or meditation class for her anxiety, which was pretty mild. When I was done explaining the plan to her, she stood up and wanted to know how much the visit would cost since she was self-pay. When I told her the price, she got mad and angrily said, "that much? But you didn't do anything!" To her way of thinking, prescriptions are the proof a doctor did something.

D. Medical equipment

Prescriptions for medical equipment join medications for those things doctors just do. A hands-on physician often has equipment around and the experience to give to the patient and train her how to use it. Some equipment requires "prior authorization" before an official approval (just as some off-label or non-"formulary" medications do, too). Again, a good doc will consider other factors such as cost, side-effects, ease-of-use, cost, and alternatives just as with medications.

E. Therapies

In the U.S., there are as many therapy companies as there are illnesses. Traditional medicine has backed away from alternative therapies that may even be effective. And those alternative therapies that were once considered placebo at best, harmful at worst, sometimes make their way into the traditional medicine armamentarium as long as the government and insurance companies pay for them. My own chiropractor is great and he is a part of the largest hospital system in southeast Wisconsin. Yoga and Tai Chi classes are often offered but I have yet to see one paid for by an insurance company. Acupuncture, too has its place.

So, what therapy to choose? Is any therapy needed at all? Is it mandatory for that particular condition? For example, physical therapy is required after knee replacement. Cognitive behavioral therapy is a great adjunct to psychiatric intervention and the two often have a synergistic effect meaning that the results they provide together outweigh the benefits alone and so are more than additive.

F. Referrals/Consultations

Adding systems to my top-to-bottom exam is not an accident. In going head-to-toe, a physician can find abnormalities throughout the exam and then needs to determine if the findings all fit together nicely to describe one diagnosis ("Occam's Razor"). Or rather does one diagnosis describe all of the symptoms (the subjective part of the note) and all of the findings (what your physician finds out about you through examination and testing).

So what to do with that knowledge? If the signs and symptoms point to a pathology that is a part of a particular system, the next step may well be to call in a specialist in that system. Is it mainly a joint or connective tissue issue? Refer to a Rheumatologist (see how the abbreviations I used previously help steer this cart into a certain direction?). Does the FH, PMH, and HPI make a doctor focus his exam onto a certain body part or system so that he needs to consult with a specialist in that system field? For example, a 22 year-old man comes in with complaints of a swollen, painful testicle. A doctor can pretty much focus on the genital system although a shout-out to the mental status is needed. How painful is it? Is the guy mildly, moderately, or severely incapacitated by the pain? Based on the history of the illness, can he be given Bactrim-DS, a pain pill, and be sent home? Or should he be referred to a GU specialist, general surgeon, or Infectious Disease (ID) specialist?

G. Follow-up

Believe it or not, how a physician addresses follow-up care with his patient is a significant part of medical decision-making. If a doc starts a patient on a new medication, when is it expected to work? When should she return to the clinic if it isn't working by then? If a patient is sent out to the laboratory or radiology department for testing, when is a follow-up scheduled in order to go over results? What is the patient to do in the meantime? What if critical lab values come back: is there a contingency plan spelled out in the charting for that?

A patient goes to see a specialist. When can the specialist see him? Based on that, when should your patient return to you to go over the specialist's findings? Will the specialist now take over care?

A patient goes to physical therapy. How long will it last or is that up to the physical therapist? What end points does the doc and patient agree on? When does the patient return to clinic ("RTC") to evaluate progress? Depending on therapy, do changes need to be made to the medications? Added? Removed? Taken differently?

Case Study: for Mrs. G's rash caused by an ocean-dwelling organism, I prescribed two medications, a topical steroid cream and Loratadine, an anti-histamine meant to decrease itching. I also advised her to buy OTC Caladryl and do it this way: apply the steroid cream first. Wait 5-10 minutes to allow it to dry and dissolve into her skin. Then apply the Caladryl lotion which not only relieves itching but also causes a barrier allowing the steroid cream to be more effective.

For her hip arthritis, I advised her to purchase ibuprofen (a NSAID) OTC and to use it in appropriate doses whenever she developed pain. For prophylaxis, I urged her to take two ibuprofen just prior to long walks with her husband. For more severe cases, she could also apply a heating pad, making sure that she does not burn her skin. I advise cold treatment for acute injuries since adding heat is like throwing gasoline on a fire. For chronic injuries, especially those like degenerative joint diseases and adhesions, I advise heat. No heat on bones that lie directly under the skin as a person could burn the bone before the skin gets burned.

The last two "therapies" involve one behavioral modification and one alternative medicine suggestion. Based on my discussions with the ER physician in Florida, I told Mrs. G to go home and boil her swimsuit in water as hot as she could. This destroys the cysts and their "hooks" that were causing her rash. They remain active for weeks after swimming and heat removes the cause.

The second suggestion was to take up yoga classes. The slow, gentle stretches of yoga increase flexibility in arthritic joints and decrease pain. Her insurance would not cover this so she would have to pay for classes herself or get a good video for home use.

SUMMARY

"There are, in truth, no specialties in medicine, since to know fully many of the most important diseases a man must be familiar with their manifestations in many organs.

---William Osler

I now give you Mrs. G's full SOAP Note. Try reading through it and see if it now makes sense. If I have done my job well, you should be able to get through it easily, making very few reference checks to the body of the book or the Glossary. As you read it, try to "think like a doctor" and imagine how all of the many small parts make up a very integrated whole.

SUBJECTIVE

Mrs. G is a 62 year-old woman who is seen for a rash that is getting worse. The rash started one week ago on the skin of her abdomen. It is very itchy. She describes the rash as "little red bumps" that have spread from her abdomen, across her lower back, and even down her pelvic region to the top of the front of her thighs.

She explains that she has used OTC Caladryl Lotion which does lessen the itching for a few hours but has failed to halt the spread of the rash. Cold water also works for itch relief but only for the duration of application.

As an aside, Mrs. G states that her right hip hurts when she walks any significant distance. The pain in her right hip occurs only after walking at least 6 city blocks. Resting makes it feel better as does taking OTC ibuprofen. Ice has no effect. The pain is described as "dull" and does not radiate anywhere else. It gets progressively worse the further she walks and can start out as low as a "4" on a scale of 0-10 and end up debilitating her when it gets to an "8". She first noticed the pain about 2 years ago, before her husband's retirement, but it is much more noticeable now that he and she spend more time walking together.

While Mrs. G states that she obviously has had rashes in the past, this is the first time for her that one has lasted this long and it is worrying her. Her only diagnosed medical condition is HTN and she takes Lisinopril once-a-day which does control her blood pressure. She has never had any serious side-effects from it and as far as she knows, does not have any drug allergies. She is allergic to ragweed but at this time of year (early spring), she has not had any problems. During allergy season, she self-medicates with OTC Loratidine, which is currently at their house in Florida.

Since her husband's retirement two years ago, the couple bought a house on the east coast of Florida. They just returned to the Midwest to visit relatives last week, about the same time as the onset of the rash. They enjoy each others company and spend their leisure time going for walks, swimming in the ocean, and eating out. Mrs. G has never felt better in her relationship with her husband and domestic violence is not now nor ever has been a concern.

She has two healthy grown children, one boy and one girl. At 45 years of age, she had a cholecystectomy to remove her gallbladder.

The same year she had an elective hysterectomy. Because her uterus was removed, she does not know precisely when she started menopause but believes she had peri-menopausal symptoms about 10 years ago.

No one else in her family has the same symptoms, including her husband. Her mother had SLE and died of complications related to a CVA at 85 years old. Her father had Type II Diabetes Mellitus, heart disease, emphysema, and died of an Acute M. I. when he was 68. Mrs. G believes that most of his problems were due to poor lifestyle choices including smoking 1-2 packs of cigarettes a day for 50 years and eating a poor diet.

The patient started smoking cigarettes when she was 15 but quit when she got pregnant with her first child at 22 years old. She does have a history of marijuana use during her "hippie days" but feels it was not an addiction. She does drink socially but cannot remember the last time she got drunk. She had been a stay-at-home mom for 30 years and once her second child left home, she volunteered at church and at a local assisted living facility. She has no known long-term exposure to any noxious chemicals "unless you count household cleaners." Up until two years ago, Mr. and Mrs. G had two cats and a dog. Since then, the dog died and the cats were given away to friends prior to going to Florida.

OBJECTIVE

Mrs. G is a well-nourished, obese female. Vital signs show a heart rate of 78 BPM, a BP of 142/88, a RR of 16/minute, and a temperature of 98.8 degrees Fahrenheit. Her height is 63 inches and her weight is 195 pounds giving her a BMI of 34.5.

Head is NCAT. Pupils are equally round and reactive to light and accommodation. EOM-I. Sclerae are white. While Mrs. G wears corrective lenses, vision was not tested.

Ears are clear bilaterally and hearing is grossly normal. No nasal discharge is present and nasal mucus membranes are moist. Pharynx is clear; uvula rises midline. Teeth show normal signs of aging but there are no obvious tooth fractures.

Neck is supple with a FROM. The posterior neck is nontender and without spasms. Palpation of the anterior neck is without thyromegaly or masses. There is no cervical lymphadenopathy.

Upper back shows mild kyphosis. Spine is otherwise midline and parathoracic muscles are without tenderness or spasms. There is no nipple retraction on visual inspection; a full breast examination is deferred.

Heart has a RRR and is without murmurs or rubs. No edema is noted.
Lungs are CTA bilaterally and there is good respiratory excursion. No cyanosis is noted.

Abdomen is obese; ND; bowel sounds are NA and present in all quadrants. Abdomen is soft and nontender to palpation. No masses or HSM. She does have a rash present on the skin of her lower abdomen. Visual inspection shows spread of her abdominal rash to her inguinal areas bilaterally. A full description of the rash is found under "DERM."

Lumbar spine is straight and non-tender. There is minor tenderness along the right paralumbar muscles but no spasms are palpable. She has limited ROM to forward flexion at the waist, limited by both an increase of pain and decreased flexibility.

Right lateral hip is tender to palpation. She has FROM of the right lower extremity at the hip with increasing pain to lateral abduction. The right anterior-superior iliac crest is elevated anteriorly about 3 cm above the left.

Of note, she does have a single right inguinal lymph node, about 1cm round, which is tender, soft, and mobile.

MSK exam shows FROM of her head and shoulders. Spine is described as above. Gait is occasionally hesitant due to pain in her right hip but otherwise normal. Grip strength in both hands is strong (+5/5) and she is able to stand on her tip-toes.

Mrs. G's skin is warm and dry; mucus membranes are moist. There is no cyanosis or edema. She has a red, papular rash from the skin of the lower quadrants of her abdomen bilaterally which radiates into both inguinal areas. Papules are 1-2mm round and raised. The patient's mucus membranes are moist and she is well-hydrated. There is no cervical lymphadenoptathy and one right inguinal lymph node and no enlarged thyroid or thyroid masses are palpable.

Mrs. G's gait is hesitant due to pain in her right hip. CNN II-XII were tested and are grossly intact. Speech has a normal cadence and reflects appropriate thought content. Balance is good and she is able to perform heel-to-toe walking without difficulty.

The patient is A, A, Ox3, and in mild distress secondary to itchiness. She is not anxious but is concerned about her illness. Her mood is appropriate to the situation, not sad, and she expresses no suicidal or homicidal ideations.

ASSESSMENT (DIAGNOSES)

1. Rash and other nonspecific skin eruption: ICD-10 R21
2. Unilateral primary osteoarthritis, right hip: ICD-10 M16.11
3. Low Back Pain: ICD-10 M54.5
4. Essential (primary) hypertension: ICD-10 I10
5. Adult (Moderate) Obesity with Body Mass Index (BMI) 34.0-34.9: ICD-10 Z68.34

PLAN

For her rash, I prescribed two medications: a topical steroid cream and Loratadine. I also advised her to buy OTC Caladryl lotion and do it this way: apply the steroid cream first. Wait 5-10 minutes to allow it to dry and dissolve into her skin, then apply the Caladryl lotion.

For her pain issues, I advised her to purchase ibuprofen OTC and to use it in appropriate doses whenever she developed pain. For prophylaxis, I urged her to take two ibuprofen just prior to long walks with her husband. For more severe cases, she could also apply a heating pad, making sure that she does not burn her skin.

I told Mrs. G to go home and boil her swimsuit in water as hot as she could. This destroys the cysts and their "hooks" that were causing her rash.

I also recommended that she consult with a yoga instructor who specializes in teaching people with health issues such as hypertension and obesity once she got back home to Florida. Yoga has also been shown to reduce blood pressure in some people, which is an added benefit.

Lastly, we discussed diet and nutrition. I went over my usual diet advice (see Additional Resources section), essential supplements, and nutrient timing.

Mrs. G is to RTC in 2 weeks to see how the therapies are working and to monitor her blood pressure. If the rash continues past 3 days after boiling her swimsuit, she should return for further re-evaluation and a possible increase in the strength of her steroid cream. She should RTC sooner if symptoms worsen, if shortness-of-breath develops, or if she develops drug intolerance (although I believe this would be low considering the safety profiles of the two prescribed medications). Use of the medications and side-effects were discussed prior to leaving the clinic for home. She left ambulatory and in good spirits.

Glossary

Medicine is full of words hardly used by non-medical people and I have done my best to highlight those words that could be new to you. It has a language of its own, a descendant of Greek, Latin, and English linguistic parents.

"Jargon" (words commonly used by a specific profession) in medicine sometimes acts as a mechanism for excluding people not familiar with the terms, but more importantly, acts as a way to express long terms and concepts succinctly. For example, "abdomen is non-distended, bowel sounds are normoactive, and there is no hepatosplenomegaly" is a lot easier to say than "his belly is not bloated, I heard bowel sounds in every area I listened to and they sounded normal, and I did not feel any enlargement of the liver or spleen."

In addition to this jargon or medspeak, medicine also has a tendency to make acronyms of almost any phrase longer than two words.

By itself, this Glossary is a good beginner's medical dictionary. See also http://www.nlm.nih.gov/medlineplus/mplusdictionary.html for an easy online medical dictionary.

Angiotensin Converting Enzyme Inhibitor (ACE-Inhibitor): A particular class of medications used for hypertension and congestive heart failure. One example is Lisinopril. They are a part of the standard post-AMI medication regime which also includes baby aspirin, a beta-blocker, and a type of cholesterol lowering medication known as a "statin."

Acute Myocardial Infarction (AMI): a heart attack or acute myocardial infarction occurs when one of the arteries that supplies the heart muscle becomes blocked. Blockage is the result of atherosclerosis with acute clot formation. The blockage results in damaged tissue and a permanent loss of contraction of this portion of the heart muscle.

Anterior Superior Iliac Crest (ASIC): top of the hips.

Assisted living facility (ALF): housing facilities for people with disabilities or the elderly. These facilities provide supervision or assistance with activities of daily living (ADLs), coordination of services by outside health care providers, and monitoring of resident activities to help to ensure their health, safety, and well-being.

Beats Per Minute (BPM): heart rate measurement. Normal range varies with age.

Bilateral: pertaining to, involving, or affecting two or both sides.

Bilaterally symmetrical: having identical parts on each side of a line drawn down the middle of the body.

Blood Pressure (BP): the pressure of the blood against the inner walls of the blood vessels, varying in different parts of the body during different phases of contraction of the heart and under different conditions of health, exertion, *etc.*

Body Mass Index (BMI): an index for assessing overweight and underweight, obtained by dividing body weight in kilograms by height in meters squared: a measure of 25 or more is considered overweight.

Cerebrovascular accident (CVA): a sudden interruption of the blood supply to the brain caused by rupture of an artery in the brain (cerebral hemorrhage) or the blocking of a blood vessel, as by a clot of blood (cerebral occlusion).

Chief Complaint (CC): The chief complaint is a brief description of why you are seeking medical attention.

Cholecystectomy: surgical removal of the gall bladder.

Demographics: the statistical data of a population, especially those showing average age, income, education, etc.

Dermatological (DERM): pertaining to the skin.

Diagnosis (Dx): "the process of determining which disease or condition explains a person's symptoms and signs. It is most often referred to as diagnosis with the medical context being implicit. The information required for diagnosis is typically collected from a history and physical examination of the person seeking medical care. Often, one or more diagnostic procedures, such as diagnostic tests, are also done during the process."

Ears, Nose, and Throat (ENT): the system (and hence the practitioners) pertaining to disorders of the ear, nose and throat, as well as, the head and neck.

Emphysema: a chronic, irreversible disease of the lungs characterized by abnormal enlargement of airspaces in the lungs accompanied by destruction of the tissue lining the walls of the air spaces.

Endocrine (ENDO): the collection of glands that secrete hormones directly into the circulatory system directed towards distant target organs. The major endocrine glands include the pineal gland,pituitary gland, pancreas, ovaries, testes, thyroid gland, parathyroid gland, and adrenal glands.

Family History (FH): part of a patient's medical history in which questions are asked in an attempt to find out whether the patient has hereditary tendencies toward particular diseases.

Focused Exam: a limited exam of the affected body area or organ system

General (GEN) Exam: A broad description of a patient on initial presentation including his or her appearance, hydration, posture, weight, and body shape.

Heart Disease: any condition of the heart that impairs its functioning.

Heart Rate (HR): the number of heartbeats per minute. The normal adult heart rate is 60-100 BPM.

Hemoglobin (Hgb or HGB): the iron-containing molecule found in red blood cells which transports oxygen from the lungs to the rest of the body.

History (Hx): a collection of information obtained from the patient and from other sources concerning the patient's physical status as well as his or her psychological, social, and sexual function.

History of Present Illness (HPI): an account obtained during the interview with the patient of the onset, duration, and character of the present illness.

Hypertension (HTN): high blood pressure. See Additional Resources section for classification of pressures.

Hysterectomy: surgical removal of the uterus.

Ideations: normal and abnormal ideas usually expressed by talking. But I have seen unusual ideas presented through mime, rhyme, and dance. Rarely, though.

Integumentary: the outer protective layer or covering of an animal, such as skin or a cuticle.

Lisinopril: an ACE-inhibiting drug (trade name Zestril) administered as an antihypertensive and after heart attacks.

Lupus or Systemic Lupus Erythematosus (SLE): a chronic autoimmune disease that can affect almost any organ system; thus, its presentation and course are highly variable.

Medical decision-making: a cognitive process for selecting a course of action in the context of health or medical diagnosis and treatment.

Menopause: the period of permanent cessation of menstruation, usually occurring between the ages of 45 and 55.

Mental Status (MS or MSE): an important part of the clinical assessment process in psychiatric practice. It is a structured way of observing and describing a patient's current state of mind, under the domains of appearance, attitude, behavior, mood and affect, speech, thought process, thought content, perception, cognition, insight and judgment.

Neurological System (Neuro): a complex, sophisticated system that regulates and coordinates body activities. It is made up of two major divisions, including the following:
1. **Central nervous system** - consisting of the brain and spinal cord.
2. **Peripheral nervous system** - consisting of all other neural elements.

Ophthalmology (OPTHO): branch of medical science dealing with the anatomy, functions, and diseases of the eye.

Ophthalmoscope: instrument for viewing the interior of the eye or examining the retina.

Organ system: a group of organs that work together for one purpose.

Otoscope: instrument for examining the external canal and tympanic membrane of the ear.

Over-the-counter (OTC): medication sold legally without a doctor's prescription.

Oxygen Saturation (SO_2): pertains to the amount of oxygen in blood and tissues. It is clinically measured using a **Pulse Oximeter**, that little light clip the nurse or MA slips onto the end of your finger. Technically, a pulse oximeter measures the amount of oxygen attached to hemoglobin in arterial blood and is written as **SaO_2.**

Pain Assessment Scale: Patients rate pain on a scale from 0-10, 0 being no pain and 10 being the worst pain imaginable. Patients who cannot verbalize/comprehend pain scales are assessed with different types of scales, such as a scale with corresponding faces depicting various levels of pain is shown to the patient and they select one. A rating is taken before administering any medication and after the specified time frame to rate the efficacy of treatment.

Papules: a well-circumscribed, raised elevated lesion of the skin. No evidence of fluid inside is visible.

Past Medical History (PMH): a narrative or record of past events and circumstances relevant to a patient's current state of health. It is an account of past diseases, injuries, treatments, and other medical facts.

Pathologies: any deviation from a healthy, normal, or efficient condition.

Peri-menopausal: Peri-menopause encompasses the years leading up to menopause, which officially starts when a woman's period has completely stopped for one year. Peri-menopause, can range from two to ten years.

Physical: the process by which a medical professional investigates the body of a patient for signs of disease.

Plan: This describes what the health care provider will do to treat the patient – ordering labs, referrals, procedures performed, medications prescribed, etc.

Post-partum: occurring after birth.

PQRST: Mnemonic for assessing pain. Provocation with movement, pressure (such as palpation) or other external factor makes the problem better or worse. Quality of the pain per the patient's description. This is the patient's description of the pain: whether it is sharp, dull, crushing, burning, tearing, or some other feeling, along with the pattern, such as intermittent, constant, or throbbing. Radiation, whether it radiates (extends) or moves to any other area. Severity of the pain usually using the pain score (usually on a scale of 0 to 10). Zero is no pain and ten is the worst pain possible.

Provocative: tending or serving to provoke; inciting, stimulating, irritating, or vexing.

Reflex: noting or pertaining to an involuntary response to a stimulus, the nerve impulse from a receptor being transmitted inward to a nerve center that in turn transmits it outward to an effector, occurring in reaction; responsive.

Respiratory Rate (RR): rate at which a person inhales and exhales; usually measured to obtain a quick evaluation of a person's health.

Social History (SH): a review of the patient's living arrangements, occupation, marital status, number of children, drug use (including tobacco, alcohol, other recreational drug use), recent foreign travel, and exposure to environmental pathogens through recreational activities.

Sphygmomanometer: instrument, often attached to an inflatable air-bladder cuff and used with a stethoscope, for measuring blood pressure in an artery.

Stethoscope: instrument used in auscultation to convey sounds in the chest or other parts of the body to the ear of the examiner.

Subjective: describes the patient's current condition in narrative form. This section usually includes the patient's chief complaint.

Type II Diabetes Mellitus (DMII): a sometimes asymptomatic form of diabetes mellitus characterized by diminished tissue sensitivity to insulin and sometimes by impaired beta cell function, exacerbated by obesity and often treatable by diet and exercise.

Uterus: the enlarged, muscular, expandable portion of the oviduct in which the fertilized ovum implants and develops or rests during prenatal development; the womb of certain mammals.

Vital signs (VS): Index of essential body functions, comprising heart rate, body temperature, and respiration. May also include Oxygen Saturation.

References

http://www.wongbakerfaces.org/

http://www.nhlbi.nih.gov/guidelines/obesity/BMI/bmicalc.htm

http://apps.who.int/classifications/icdReferences

http://www.wongbakerfaces.org/

http://www.nhlbi.nih.gov/guidelines/obesity/BMI/bmicalc.htm

http://apps.who.int/classifications/icd10/browse/2010/en#/XII

https://ocm.ama-assn.org/OCM/CPTRelativeValueSearch.do

http://www.cms.gov/Regulations-and-Guidance/Legislation/CLIA/Certificate_of_-Waiver_Laboratory_Project.html

http://www.nlm.nih.gov/medlineplus/mplusdictionary.html

http://www.amazon.com/Medical-Decision-Making-Hal-Sox/dp/1930513798

http://www.smdm.org

http://www.cms.gov/Medicare/CMS-Forms/CMS-Forms/CMS-Forms-List.html

Additional Resources

Body Mass Index for adults aged 18-65 years old (Percent)

Very Severely Underweight: 15 and below

Severely Underweight: 15-15.9

Underweight: 16-18.4

Healthy Weight: 18.5-24.9

Overweight: 25-34.9

Moderately Obese: 30-34.9

Severely Obese: 35-39.9

Very Severely Obese = "Morbid Obesity": 40 and above

Blood Pressure Classifications (mmHg)

Normal: 90-119/60-79

Prehypertension: 120-139/80-89

Stage 1 HTN: 140-159/90-99

Stage 2 HTN: >159/>100

Oxygen Saturation (SaO$_2$)

Normal (Pulse Oximeter): 95 to 100 percent.

Values under 90 percent are considered low.

Dr. Mangold's Diet and Supplement Advice

1. Eat low on the Glycemic Index ("GI")

2. Avoid gluten

3. The less processed the food, the better

4. Eat or drink a probiotic every day or take a probiotic supplement at Least once-a-day

5. Take a multivitamin ("MVI") at least every day, with food

6. Unless contraindicated, supplement with fish oil or krill oil

7. Other recommended supplements: Vitamin C, Vitamin D, Vitamin E, and a Vitamin B Complex

http://upwardsbound.blogspot.com

http://www.physiciansoapnotes.com

http://www.wikihow.com/Write-a-Soap-Note

http://www.emednotes.com/eMedNotesExampleNote.pdf

http://www.ttuhsc.edu/som/fammed/ttmedcast/ttmedcast_soapnote.html

http://www.soapnoteapp.com/

http://archivists.metapress.com/content/d54gn70748865222/10/browse/2010/en#/XII

https://ocm.ama-assn.org/OCM/CPTRelativeValueSearch.do

http://www.cms.gov/Regulations-and-Guidance/Legislation/CLIA/Certificate_of_-Waiver_Laboratory_Project.html

http://www.nlm.nih.gov/medlineplus/mplusdictionary.html

http://www.amazon.com/Medical-Decision-Making-Hal-Sox/dp/1930513798

http://www.smdm.org

http://www.cms.gov/Medicare/CMS-Forms/CMS-Forms/CMS-Forms-List.html

Books by Michael Mangold MD

How To Think Like a Doctor

Cómo Pensar Como un Doctor

Barefoot Doctors 2

Mythomania: A Psychodrama

My Worst Thanksgiving Ever: A PanAmerican Tragedy

Mi Peor Acción de Gracias Siempre

Desperately Seeking Cereal: A Travelogue

Worst Thanksgiving Ever Trilogy

About the Author

Michael Mangold M.D. is a doctor, educator, and father of many. After graduating from Rosalind Franklin University of Health Sciences/ Chicago Medical in 1990, he embarked on a 23 year career in primary care medicine including 15 years as an Emergency Physician. His medical interests include wilderness and travel medicine, addictionology, and trauma psychology. Recently, he has turned his attentions to education and and teaching students through the internet.

Winding down his career as an ER physician, Dr. Mangold went to Nicaragua in 2013 to teach medical English to the med students in

Puerto Cabezas. His plans changed though, when the medical director of the school could not obtain funding so he was forced to look for other sources of income in Managua first, then San Juan del Sur, his adopted home. While in SJdS, Dr. Mangold published three eBooks: How to Think Like a Doctor, Cómo Pensar Como un Doctor, and Barefoot Doctors. He wrote all three with the intention of bringing quality medical knowledge and practice to underserved areas of the world.

His mission was cut short over the Thanksgiving weekend that year when he was mugged five times that Thursday and Friday night. By the fifth mugging he was left for dead. Why would any sane gringo be out after dark in a large Central American city? He was trying to find his son Ben, who (as he later found out) was being hidden by the American embassy there. Find the full story in his book, <u>My Worst Thanksgiving Ever: A PanAmerican Tragedy</u> and its prequel, <u>Mythomania: A Psychodrama</u>.

<u>Desperately Seeking Cereal</u> is the sequel to "Worst Thanksgiving." It is the fourth installment in his "Bridges Series" and it documents events that occurred around the holiday season in and around León, Nicaragua. He is concurrently writing a screenplay, "Elkton Rules: the Little Prison That Thought it Could" and the follow-up to "Cereal," <u>Starting From Spat</u>.

Dr. Mangold's main emphasis these days is in democratizing Medicine: bringing the knowledge and wisdom of this science and art into the hands of everyone who can use them. For after all, (as Dr. Paul Farmer says) "this could be very simple: the well should take care of the sick."

You can find Michael Mangold on Twitter @thanksgivingD12 and on Facebook at facebook.com/mkmangold

Dr. Mangold blogs about health and medicine at www.upwardsbound.blogspot.com

Printed in Great Britain
by Amazon